The Color Of Seizures

Kate Taylor
Jeffrey Underwood, RN

The Color of Seizures

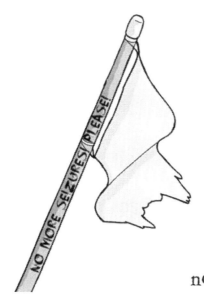

Brain buzzes
beseige my
balance...
Seizure
strikes and I am
shaken. The
white flag raised.
I surrender yet
again. Please,
no more seizures!

Kate Taylor

Jeffrey Underwood, RN

The Color Of Seizures

Kate Taylor Jeffrey Underwood, RN

ISBN-10: 1515243052

ISBN-13: 978-1515243052

Acknowledgments

Jeffrey Underwood, RN

You are much more than a co-author to me. As a registered nurse, your wealth of knowledge, wisdom, and the kindness you show towards me and the challenge of PNES that I face are all invaluable to me. Even more so, the caring love that you give me affects me always in body, mind, and spirit. You know you have a permanent place in my heart.

Lorna Myers, PhD
Director
PNES Diagnostic and Treatment Program

Dr. Myers, you introduced me to PNES. I will forever be grateful for those words that spell acceptance for me.

My Doctors and Therapists

Your respect for me and the support that you give me are crucial to my well-being.

Family and Friends

All my loved ones, you hold me up like no one else can.

All those who are challenged by PNES

United we share the feelings of hope and peace.

Introduction

Before I was diagnosed with non-epileptic seizures, most nights, I awoke with that worms-crawling-in-my-legs feeling, and many nights I awoke with my right leg and arm thrashing about the bed. My head twisted to the left and I was afraid I might not be able to breathe. When the movement stopped, I got out of bed and paced the floor for the rest of the night, worrying. I was terrified; even more terrified when it happened to me at work at the oddest of times. I recall that someone had laughed and said that I had gone over the rainbow. It wasn't funny then and the remembrance isn't funny now.

My closest friends from work brought me to the emergency room where I was poorly treated. I was admitted and given enough medication that caused me to totally black out for five days. I recall absolutely nothing.

While I was in the hospital I underwent both an MRI and a CT scan. Both tests appeared normal, but I appeared anything but normal.

The diagnosis was made. It stated that I was having pseudo seizures and that I was crying out for help. I was wide awake when I heard those words.

My entire body dropped and I emotionally wrapped my arms around myself. I agree. I was crying out for help. I was begging for relief from my pain. I was pleading to know what was wrong with me. I was imploring them to put an end to these seizures. Fear, like a wound, opened up inside my spirit.

I was out of work on medical leave for five months.

The seizures continued. I suffered depression deep enough to nearly drown in a well of pain.

I was evaluated by a neuropsychologist with whom I spent an entire day. I will be doing the same again soon.

I saw and still see my therapist regularly. I also saw my psychiatrist and continue to seek her care regularly. I take medication daily for these seizures.

It was when I was poking around on the internet to try and find some information that would provide details about the seizures that I finally found an answer. I stumbled upon a site, PNES, Psychological Non Epileptic Seizures, where I felt welcomed by Lorna Myers, PhD.

As I read, Dr. Myers explained that seizures such as mine that did not appear to be epilepsy were called psychogenic non-epileptic seizures, also known as PNES. To finally have an appropriate name for my condition exhilarated me! I was so relieved to finally give it a name! I bought her book, "Psychogenic Non-epileptic Seizures: A Guide" and I read it from beginning to end and I understood my condition.

I bought several copies to give to my loved ones, my therapist, my psychiatrist, and my primary care physician. The therapist and the psychiatrist understood well. My family and friends would come to understand. And, maybe my doctor would too.

What I am sure of is that this condition is treatable. While I continue to have seizures, I know that I am not crazy and that I will be okay.

However, while giving the seizures the name PNES helped me immensely, my reaction to every seizure then and every seizure since… I HATE THEM!

I hate the shaking. I hate the jerking, bending, and twisting. I hate the crying. I hate the swearing. I hate the burning pain and spasms.

My body, mind, and spirit continue to cry out, but this time for loving support.

I have a special person in my life who gives me love, support, encouragement, and who cares about me enough to be honest with me when I need that as well.

I am surrounded by the acceptance and love from my family and friends.

There's something comforting though when persons with any like condition come together with others who share the same issues.

That is how "The Color of Seizures" came to be.

Between front and back cover, this book is a place to go to in order to find loving support. It is a place to begin to find well-being. It is a place to be with others who withstand the challenges that these non-epileptic seizures bring. "The Color of Seizures" offers those with PNES a chance to find balance.

Being healthy encompasses all our parts, not just our physical body. When our emotions are in turmoil or our mind is bombarded with obsessive thoughts our health is compromised and we already know the result: seizures. It is important to create balance in our lives by nurturing our entire selves. It is paramount to our total health to meet our spiritual, mental, emotional, and physical needs.

If we feel balanced, we will experience joy in what we do. We will have a sense of purpose and feel that our lives have meaning. We will treat ourselves with love and respect. We will also be loving and respectful with our loved ones. We will feel calm and less stressed and anxious. That can lead to a quieting of our seizures.

Within the pages of "The Color of Seizures" you will find interactive activities. The activities are simple, inexpensive, and fun ways to make a connection with you.

There are reflective questions which are opportunities to examine and express your emotions and feelings.

The Personal Three Day Retreat that follows is a guide to give you an opportunity for quiet self-care. It is designed to be uniquely your own experience. The guide is only that - you will find suggestions and opportunities for your own choices towards wellness.

Together, we say as a community of friends:
PNES... Finally, it has a name!
We are comforted and comfortable.
We feel acceptance.
We are not alone.
It is not the end.

Be blessed with healing in your body, mind, and spirit.

May your seizures be quieted.

Contents

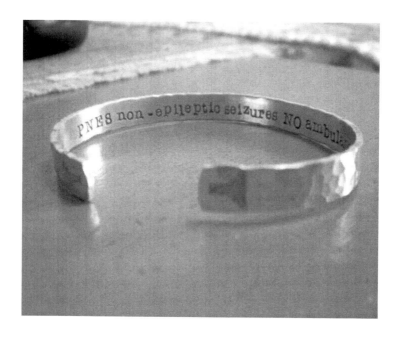

Chapter 1 Rag Rugs and Backstories

When times were lean, careful settler women were forced into repurposing materials. Nothing went to waste. Ragged clothes, old woolen shirts, a shirtwaist dress faded and threadbare, any type of cloth really, all torn into strips became the weft for weaving the rugs. What emerged from the work of moving old cloth in and out of the warp strings to be tugged hard on by the loom, tightening them all together into one piece, was something durable, even beautiful, to look at. Often, as a child, I'd lie on the floor and peek into the materials in the rag rugs that we had and make up stories about each color and pattern of cloth.

Sometimes I feel like an unfinished rag rug, still in the loom. Pieces of my life, torn into long strips, tied together, and wound into a ball are poised to intertwine with the spirit; that spirit which becomes the weaver that tugs the warp that tightens and holds me together. Some days, well, many days, I don't see the beauty of the strips that have been woven together already.

Each of us has a backstory. Our own history underlies and leads us to the situation that is going on in our life right now. It is our personal history, rich with every single event in our life that affects how we came to have PNES, psychogenic non-epileptic seizures, how we live with that condition today, and how we will live with it through many tomorrows.

My personal backstory is so filled with tattered, ragged bits of cloth that my rag rug will be carpet sized when I am finished.

There is so much that happened in my life from the time that I was born, it caused me to write a book. Even the title of the book, "The Pink Eraser", refers to a traumatic experience that I had when I was in kindergarten. I have memories from as early as the age of two years.

I lived once again through the events of my life as I wrote the novel. I had been in the deep well of depression for so long. I was stuck and couldn't move. I cried out asking for help. People yelled for me to come out of that well. They tossed ropes of rescue down to pull me up. They encouraged me to make the climb, telling me how to do it. When I tried with their aid, I fell back down, deeper into the muck that was dank, thick, and musty. Finally, they gave up and walked away. I stopped crying out. What could I do? If I wanted to be free I had to climb out on my own; one slippery, muddy brick at a time. I slipped a couple of times, but eventually I saw the top and tumbled out onto solid earth and found myself in puddles of sunshine. I knew the well was there and I looked at it once in a while, but I didn't go near it. Eventually, I moved far away from the well.

I forget where it is now.

The details of my childhood are many. Listing all of them won't add any strength to the telling of my backstory for now. Those facts of my early years of development into my adult years are a ball of rags; many colors wound and already pulled tightly through my rug. However, some of the backstory that happened to me as an adult and how I got into the well are important for me to share. Each of us knows fully the details of our lives, some similar to others, most unique to us only.

A troubled family, plus high anxiety, plus stress, plus codependency, as well as the addition of even more signs and symptoms, all equal PNES for me.

My life with PNES is not a ball wound from black and grey rags. It's a rather large ball, a shade of soft faded red. Bright enough to stand out but the shade doesn't steal the eye away from the other colors and demand all the attention. The torn rags are shorter than the others, so that they are woven in smaller pieces throughout the rag rug that is my life. I am grateful for the spirit that I call my Higher Power who is the weaver of my life. The colors and designs in the rug being woven of and for me are held tightly together. My life will be a carpet of many various colors one day. The red will be interspersed throughout and I will know the why of its color.

****

What's your back story?

Are you in the well of your own feelings? You just might decide to make the climb out. It's okay. Solid ground as well as rays and puddles of sunshine await you.

Maybe you have a basket filled with the wound colors of the cloth that has been torn into tattered and fringed rags waiting to be woven into your personal rag rug.

What color are the rag strips of PNES within your own rag rug? Express yourself in any form of color: paint, crayon, etc.

The color of my PNES...

Chapter 2 Over The Rainbow And Waiting

The Lady Who Waited

Once upon a time there was a lady who waited. She had waited for sleep for a long time. Sleep wasn't easily found. When she slept, she slept less than two hours for most nights and in that short amount of time she didn't find rest. Most nights, she would be awakened with that worms-crawling-in-her-legs feeling. Many nights she awoke with her right leg and arm thrashing about the bed. Her head twisted to the left and she was afraid she might not be able to breathe. When it stopped, she got out of bed and paced the floor for the rest of the night, worrying. She was so very afraid. It happened to her at work at the oddest of times. Someone laughed and said that she had gone over the rainbow. There were no star wishes and it took more than a lemon drop to melt her troubles.

Maybe if she waited a little longer she wouldn't go over the rainbow again. Maybe. So she waited but she went over the rainbow again and again.

She couldn't wait much longer. Every time it happened, the shaking and twisting and the burning were making her see stars and making her feel sick. So she called the doctor and waited on the phone. The receptionist told her that there was a wait for appointments, so she should wait at home by the phone until someone called her. The lady hung up the phone and waited.

The nurse called and told the lady to wait a little longer while she told the doctor. The lady continued to wait. While she waited, she felt dizzy and nauseous and the shaking came again and her head twisted too far to the left. But, she waited anyhow. After a wait, the nurse called back and said, "The doctor said that you need urgent care. Don't wait any longer. Go right to the emergency room." The lady didn't wait and did what the doctor ordered. The lady met a very nice receptionist and two very nice volunteers at the emergency room. They were kind to her while she waited.

And waited. And waited some more.

A nurse came out and called her name. The lady went into the examining area and waited a bit. The nurse, a tall woman with a firm voice, came in and wrote down on a paper towel pulled from the holder what the lady said. Then the nurse took the lady's vital signs and told the lady to get undressed and wait for the doctor. The lady felt dizzy and sick while she waited some more. Her foot began that familiar twitching before her body shook. She begged God to make it stop. God apparently wanted her to tough it out while waiting.

Just then, the doctor came in. He had a funny name. He folded his arms and leaned against the counter as he watched her shake and twist. He touched his index finger to his lips and his brow furrowed. He listened as she began to cry and to say "shit and fuck" without control. When she stopped, he asked the lady what she wanted him to do. The lady said through tears that made mascara run in rivulets down her cheeks, "Please find out what is wrong with me. This happens to me again and again. What is going on?! I shake and twist and burn in pain. I see stars, get dizzy, and feel very sick." The doctor looked in the lady's eyes. He made her touch her nose, say ABC's and stick out her tongue just like she supposed a sobriety test would be administered. He didn't touch her at all. She waited, thinking that he might do that.

The doctor told her to wait and a nurse would come and take some blood.

The nurse did come and she did take some blood.

And the waiting began again.

Waiting. Waiting. Waiting.

It seemed like a very long time that this lady was waiting. The doctor returned and said, "You appear to be anxious. Yes, I suppose anxiety caused all of what I am seeing here. I suggest that you take this medicine and wait for a few days to see if the anxiety gets better. If, in a few days, you are not better, call your PCP. You understand that's your primary care doctor. Tell him that you are still anxious even with this medication. He might prescribe more or something else entirely. You can get dressed now and wait for the nurse."

The lady dressed and waited and waited and waited.

Finally, the nurse came in and spoke gently to the lady. The nurse was a man this time; he was a very kind nurse. But, he too, had to tell the lady to wait.

The lady dressed, left the emergency room, and then went home to wait and see what would happen to the anxiety that the doctor who didn't touch her thought she had.

What do you think happened?

Yup, she still has that familiar toe tapping, wrist shaking twitch that warns her there will be no waiting before the shaking and twisting and swearing and crying will begin. She is still waiting for the shaking and twisting, the dizziness and sick feeling to get better. She's waiting for them to go away.

Waiting for things to change. Waiting for sleep.

She's back, but she's not in Kansas now. And... She's still waiting for the happy ending.

She is tired of waiting.

Yet she is still waiting beyond belief that she should have to wait anymore.

Not the End.

Kate Taylor

I was four years old when I spent three months in a hospital, fighting a kidney disease. I don't remember much except being yelled at for climbing shelves in the toy room. I don't remember much except for having to take a bath with another patient in some black tarry smelling water. I wonder if anything happened that I cannot remember.
I was five years old, attending kindergarten, when I had a traumatic experience with a teacher and my pink eraser. I felt even before that situation that I must be perfect in order to be loved. I knew it following that event. That trauma would last my entire life.

There are times during my childhood that abusive things happened. Times I remember; times I would rather forget. There was the time right after I turned 16 that I was raped on the beach. I remember saying, "No." I remember that night well.

I remember many good years of being married and having children. Those were mostly good memories, but stress, anxiety, depression, and some remembered but needing to be left unsaid memories entered in. The memories are there but remain better left unsaid.

When I was thirty-one years old, I was both anxious and frightened when I had the interior portion of the lower half of my left breast removed because I had one tumor that could be seen through my clothes from across the room. There were other tumors but I was lucky and they were benign.

Just before Christmas, when I was thirty-four years old, I had surgery for uterine cancer. I was frightened and anxious again, but returned home on Christmas Eve feeling very fortunate as all was incised successfully. I remember it was my best Christmas ever.

As an adult child of a father who abused both alcohol and me, I held the stress, anxiety, and fear inside as I tried to be the good daughter and maintain a relationship with him. Everyone has stress at work. My overwhelming sensitivity and heightened emotional state made my feelings of stress and anxiety worsen. I worked too many hours which exhausted me.

All of the signs and symptoms, shaken in a brown paper bag, caused me to develop severe and crippling insomnia. I was treated with antidepressants. That was when the restless legs started. Every night they would come and I would wrestle with them to try and sleep. About that time was when the shaking and thrashing began.

What would later be diagnosed as seizures was diagnosed as serotonin syndrome and all the antidepressants stopped and were added to the list of medicines I am allergic to.

I had many sleepless nights over two years. They were fraught with the events that caused the questions: What was going on?! What was happening to me?!

I remember the very first time that an episode happened at work. I was sitting in the chapel at work attending Mass. My right knee began to bob up and down and my heel lifted and tapped on the floor. Within seconds my entire leg was moving and my foot appeared as if I was tap dancing with one foot only. My right wrist began to tremble until my whole arm was involved. My head twisted to the left and I could not move my neck. For what seemed an hour, but was probably nearer two minutes, I continued this dance. I had no clue what had happened to me that left me to feel so lousy.

These episodes continued at home. At work when they happened and I had a near fall, staff would catch me in a wheelchair. They even occurred on the street occasionally. I managed to sit on a stone wall once and a friend who saw what was happening stopped her car, sat with me, and then gave me a ride home.

The events kept happening and happening. One day at work when I had several of the episodes, my friends took charge and transported me to the ER. Even the nurses there acted as if I was drug seeking. I was admitted to the hospital and given enough Ativan that I blacked out for five days.

I was and would later, for quite some time and even today, be treated like I was crazy.

I was out of work for five months on medical leave. When I returned, I remained in the department in which I worked but I was replaced by someone and I worked in a lesser capacity.

I would wait further to get my challenges sorted out.

****

Did you have to wait? Did you have to wait to be listened to, wait to be cared for, maybe even cared about?

Are you still waiting? Are you waiting for answers? Are you waiting for the seizures to stop?

Express your thoughts. What is it that you are waiting for?

_____

_____

_____

_____

_____

_____

_____

_____

_____

_____

_____

It Has A Name

Friends, close friends, from near and far decide it is time.

No explanation needed they see it written on my face -

Get in the car now!

Shaking, head aching, toes tapping, foot banging!

Help me! This is no show, writing now illegible words, mind screaming!

I can't make this happen! What is happening?! What is happening?!!

Onlookers ask and ask and ask. Are they testing with their questions?!

"You ladies are enabling her," admonishes the nurse with pinched face.

Dr. DoNoHarm, "Your head hurts? Poor you.

Do you want a Tylenol or Morphine?"

Patronizing ass, a Tylenol works just fine. I am not drug seeking.

But you sir, find yourself reported.

Knowing friends hurl darts of advocacy

And reach out to me with eyes full of love.

Lightbulbs of thoughtfulness brighten the close cubicle.

Curlicue of pink tubing decorates my hand and I watch the first sip of red speed up the straw.

Who am I feeding?

*Again it starts-Thumb wiggles. Arm tingles. Leg bends and
shouts*

Why???!!!!

Over and over my thoughts are interrupted abruptly.

I am in pain! Muscles growing and stretching, contracting

And banging in more directions

Than has even been intended!

Again and again! Is there no relief?!

For days, black, black, black, black, black, five in all. I know

Nothing though I see and taste, smell and feel and hear.

Yet I am not really here. Where am I while I am away?

My memory is an erased and washed clean blackboard.

Instead of sleep, the nights are filled with pacing, fear,

And repeats of muscular torment and torture.

More than two years pass by.

And now I pick up the chalk and lift my trembling hand

To write the lesson for this new day: Hope,

PNES... Finally, it has a name!

I am comforted and comfortable.

Acceptance.

Kate Taylor

Chapter 3 It Has A Name

Little chunks, no nibbles, of time are all that I can remember of my hospital stay.

I know that my friends were there. They had told me that they wouldn't leave me and I believed them, so I know they were beside me. At least, I think they were.

My family had to have been there as well. Of course, I just don't remember is all.

Was it a brief ten minute visit that changed my life forever? Something that important should be burned into my synapses, but I cannot remember. Is that one of many events that has been buried in the color of wood-burned charcoal that is lodged in the back of my brain?

I used the bathroom, bathed, got dressed, I ate, and more.

I underwent test after test.

I slept; at least I think I knew the condition of body and mind which for most people recurs nightly. My consciousness was suspended. My eyes, I am sure, were closed. My nervous system was inactive and my muscles relaxed. I don't know. It had been so long since I had closed my eyes for more than two hours, maybe I couldn't identify what sleep was. Most nights for nearly two years I would rub my eyes, stare into dark space, nod off and jerk awake. I was so fatigued in body, mind, and spirit. Even if my sleep in the hospital was drug induced, it was still sleep.

How long was my hospital stay?

I know a friend took me to stay with her for a couple nights. She had a gathering of friends, so they tell me. But where was I? Was it in my charcoal black place?

I remember having heard sounds in one open speck of time.

I couldn't see. I was in the blackened place but I had heard the banging.

I know that I was on that movable table that slid into the tube. Did someone talk to me during the procedure? Even if the procedure wasn't painless, I had no inkling of what was happening to me. Within the slice, after slice, after paper thin slice, would they find the fire colored areas that marked seizures?

I certainly didn't need a sedative to calm me or to help me from feeling claustrophobic during the procedure. In my state of exhaustion and my drug induced near unconsciousness, I only recall the bang, bang, bang.

The MRI appeared normal. The CT scan appeared normal. However, I appeared anything but normal.

The diagnosis was pseudo seizures and that I was crying out for help.

I was awake when I heard that. I was wide awake.

Ah, yes...pseudo seizures:
Pseudo /ˈsjuːdəʊ/ soo-doh.
Adjective- (informal) not genuine; pretended.
Pseudo-combining form:
1. False, pretending, or unauthentic: pseudo-intellectual.
2. Having a close resemblance to.
Word origin - from Greek pseudēs false, from pseudein to lie.

My entire body dropped and I emotionally wrapped my arms around myself. I agree; I was crying out for help. I was begging for relief from my pain. I was pleading to know what was wrong with me. I implored them to put an end to these seizures. Fear, like a wound, opened up inside my spirit.

However, my seizures are not false. I did not pretend to tremble, shake my right side violently, twist my head, and breathe too fast. My rapid heartbeat was genuine. I didn't lie. I even tried to recreate the movements that would become a seizure. I couldn't.

I felt like others thought I must be a lunatic. I was ashamed. I even considered for a while that maybe I was indeed crazy. Whatever was written in my chart by my primary care physician led others to treat me like I was non-compos mentis.

There was one time that I suffered seizure after seizure, seventeen in all. A loved one brought me to the emergency room. I continued to seize. They became unbearable and my head was screaming in pain. I had my hands over my eyes and through anguished tears stated that I had an extreme headache. On a pain scale, I would have rated it an eight. The pain was unbearable and my fear was palpable. I asked again and again for pain relief. The nurse who was sympathetic called for the doctor. He pressed his lips together, rolled his eyes and with an exasperated sigh literally brought his face within inches of mine and in a sing-song voice, "Oh, you have a headache? Would you like a Tylenol or do you want morphine?" I thought, "What the hell!?" Tylenol would be just fine. I was having a headache. I laid my arm across my eyes and I waited for medication.

Now I was drug seeking? Apparently this doctor, with both a condescending and snide attitude towards me, thought so. I reported him later for his treatment of me. I was told later that most of the emergency room doctors were not invested in the hospital, so there was no need to really care. It was evident that this particular doctor did not care.

I was out of work on medical leave for five months. The seizures continued. I suffered depression deep enough to nearly drown in a well of pain.

I saw and still see my therapist regularly. I also saw my psychiatrist and continue to seek her care regularly. I take medication daily for these seizures.

I was evaluated by a neuropsychologist with whom I spent an entire day. I had a mild seizure in the middle of the testing which in his report he noted that I appeared to have some uncontrolled movements.

Months went by before I went to see my primary care doctor. I avoided him like the plague. I practiced over and over what I would say to him when I saw him. I couldn't tolerate hearing him repeat the words once again, "Pseudo seizures and crying out for help." I couldn't tolerate knowing whatever else he might write in my chart. It was when an emergency appointment with him was clearly unavoidable that I had to see him.

When he entered the examination room and said, "Well hello," with a cheerful smile, I stopped him. I spoke quietly yet firmly. I had no time to rehearse what I said. The words flew from my mouth spontaneously.

"Don't talk to me. Don't look at me. Don't touch me until I have said what I have to say. Sit down."

His brows knit together as he sat down and responded, "Okay."

I maintained eye contact with him through tears that I couldn't control. I said what I needed to say. I spoke my truth.

"Whatever you wrote in my chart has caused other doctors and even nurses to treat me poorly. I don't even want to know what you wrote. What you write in charts clearly affects the care of your patients. Others may take what you have written in my and other patients' charts as god-speak, but you are not God and neither am I."

He asked me if he should apologize. I responded, "No. What I want you to do is to be aware of the words that you write. Be aware of how your patients feel and how they will be affected."

He did apologize. He said that he understood. I wonder what he wrote in my chart that day. I still wonder if he understands.

The seizures continued. My supportive therapist and psychiatrist helped me to understand that these episodes did not fit clearly the diagnosis of epilepsy. Anti-seizure medication helped to quell most of the seizures, yet I was afflicted then and am still afflicted with the seizures today.

It was when I was poking around on the internet to try and find some information that would provide details about the seizures that I finally found an answer. I stumbled upon a site, PNES, Psychological Non Epileptic Seizures, where I felt welcomed by Lorna Myers, PhD.

As I read, Dr. Myers explained that seizures such as mine that did not appear to be epilepsy were called psychogenic non-epileptic seizures, also known as PNES. To finally have an appropriate name for my condition exhilarated me! I was so relieved to finally give it a name! I bought her book, "Psychogenic Non-epileptic Seizures: A Guide" and I read it from beginning to end and I understood my condition.

I bought several copies to give to my loved ones, my therapist, my psychiatrist, and my primary care physician. The therapist and the psychiatrist understood well. My family and friends would come to understand. And, maybe my doctor would too. I am still not sure of his thoughts there.

What I am sure of is that this condition is treatable. While I continue to have seizures, I know that I am not crazy and that I will be okay.

How does it feel to know that you are not crazy?
That you have PNES?
That you will be okay?

It feels like a gift.

Do you want more information? Visit:

http://www.nonepilepticseizures.com/

and you will be welcomed by Lorna Myers, PhD too.

Chapter 4 Before, During, and After

This chapter is interactive and provides an opportunity for you to write your thoughts as they come to you while reading.

What are the antecedents to your seizures? What are the triggers?

Before

The reasons for the onset of PNES seizures are as unique as we who have them.
For many of us, the seizures came out of the blue without any seemingly significant cause. We may not have recognized the initial events as seizures. However, some of us may find that we have issues in common, those which could set off our seizures.

I recall at times years ago being agitated and in a state of confusion. Along with those feelings, I was restless and nauseous, my heartbeat was rapid, and I endured mild tremors all the way to violent shaking. My primary care physician at that time diagnosed me with serotonin syndrome and my depression medication was immediately discontinued. My list of allergies now includes any selective serotonin reuptake inhibitors (SSRI's), which includes many medications for depression.

Some of us have developed PNES as a result of negative life events. Nine out of ten of us have had traumatic life events that have precipitated our seizures.

Traumatic events can include the following:

Experiences like injuries, accidents, being a victim of abuse or any crime. Rape or meeting a previous abuser is a traumatic experience. Even surgical procedures, giving birth, and undergoing anesthetics can be traumatic for some. Other events such as the death of or separation from family members or friends, relationship difficulties and legal action, even job loss or natural disasters, are considered traumatic events.

I have several of the above that can be added to my personal journal, along with what happened to me in kindergarten with a pink eraser. It is my earliest memory of traumatic experiences in my life. Do not exclude events simply because of their oddity.

****

Look back at your own history. Jot down any experiences that you consider to be traumatic, even if you think that others may not agree with your interpretation of the event.

_____

_____

_____

_____

_____

_____

_____

_____

_____

_____

_____

_____

_____

_____

_____

_____

_____

_____

_____

Stress and dilemmas: Psychogenic seizures may also develop

when people face difficult choices, dilemmas that cause much stress. People sometimes talk of unspeakable dilemmas because the hard choices, which can contribute to PNES, may be difficult to discuss with others.

In an unspeakable dilemma, a person experiences himself or herself trapped in a forced choice in which there are dreaded consequences, regardless of which decision is made.

Moreover, the individual feels that the very existence of the dilemma must be kept hidden from important persons involved in the situation. For instance, someone may feel duty-bound by religious or traditional beliefs to stay in an abusive relationship although they cannot cope with the consequences of allowing the abuse to continue. Some choices may be so difficult to think about or admit to that not even the person facing the choice is fully aware of their dilemma. Therapists, psychiatrists, doctors, and even loved ones may have to point out the dilemma to the person suffering.

****

Have you faced or are you facing an unspeakable dilemma in your life? Write about it.

_____

_____

_____

_____

_____

_____

_____

_____

_____

_____

Trigger

Trigger is a term used to describe something that brings on the seizures within seconds to hours, even a week or more after.

Triggers can be cumulative.

Many of us who experience non-epileptic seizures are aware of the triggers that lead up to most of our seizures.

Triggers may involve:

Emotions- Our PNES can be triggered by emotions such as feeling stressed, upset, or anxious.
Bodily sensations- Physical symptoms can also trigger seizures. Feeling ill, having lost sleep, or feeling emotionally and physically exhausted can be significant for triggering the seizures.

Sensations- Some of us have an awareness of external triggers such as crowded places, flashing lights, or other visual impressions.

Experiences- PNES can also be triggered by certain individual experiences. Going to the doctor, attending funerals, even an evaluation or meeting with someone at work can be a stressful experience that might trigger a seizure.

Psychiatric conditions- Sometimes PNES develops as a symptom of conditions such as depression, anxiety, post-traumatic stress disorder (PTSD), or bipolar disorder.

My seizures typically start with triggers of acute stress and exhaustion. I know that when my stress level mounts to an explosive level and my sleep time plummets to near nothing, I can expect to have a seizure. Ironically, my seizures themselves rarely occur in the middle of the mess of stress and exhaustion. My body and mind wait until all is quiet and then the seizures come unexpectedly.

****

What are the triggers for your seizures?

During

What does it feel like to have non-epileptic attacks?
Most of us who experience PNES are aware of warning signs prior to the seizure's obvious manifestations. These are actually part of the seizure complex.

Warning signs may include feelings of panic, bodily symptoms such as a twitching or a preliminary movement. It may possibly include sensory symptoms which involve tasting, hearing, smelling, seeing, and feeling in some unique way. Some of us even feel removed from ourselves or the situation that we are in.

Most of us experience some degree of loss of control or awareness during our seizures. About one half of people with PNES are completely unaware during their attacks. Many of us are aware of what is going on around us but we are unable to respond. Some of us carry out activities during the seizure such as moving about or talking to others only to find that we cannot remember any of the actions later. Some people even hear or see things during the seizures which are not actually happening at the time.

Interestingly we may feel physical symptoms of panic, such as trembling, sweating, or a racing heartbeat during seizures without feeling anxious.

My warning signs may include a headache that I feel upon waking. It isn't eliminated with Ibuprofen or Tylenol. I am alerted to a twitching in my right ankle and a tiny twitch, rarely noticed by others, in my right wrist. When most of my seizures happen I usually have enough warning time to verbally alert others.

One time, a seizure occurred on an airplane just as my daughter and I, along with a plane full of passengers, were taxiing down the tarmac to take off. All the flight attendants were strapped in. My daughter was seated to my right and a male stranger to my left. I took my daughter's wrist and touched the man's hand long enough to say, "I'm going to have a seizure. I'm okay." My daughter guided him throughout my seizure. He must have been a nervous wreck!

Passengers across the aisle were aware also. I was conscious, but out of physical control.

All I could think at the onset was, "Oh my god! What if they yell for help?! What if they stop the plane?!"

The poor man! He was relieved that I could tell him. He said that he felt badly because he couldn't help. The folks across the aisle waited for me after we landed to make sure that I was okay. The woman said, "At first I thought that you were afraid of flying and then I realized that you were having a seizure." I will always remember her kindness.

When my seizures come, I typically have them in clusters. One seizure lasts for near two minutes, settles down for about thirty seconds or so, another one starts and follows suit, and then another. About thirty minutes to an hour later I will have the final seizure and the event subsides. It's exhausting! The seizures can repeat several times over the next days or week or more until they settle down.

During my seizures, my entire right side is involved with rapid hard tapping up and down, like marching in my leg. My arm thrashes about; my right wrist and hand shake vigorously back and forth. My head twists too far to the left and I cannot move my neck. My breathing is rapid and I usually cry and swear. I can hear others but, in the throes of the seizure, I cannot respond.

****

What warning signs do you experience?

_____

_____

_____

_____

_____

_____

Describe in detail what happens to you during a seizure.

Many people find it frightening to witness us having a seizure. It is important to plan ahead if you can and tell people who may see you have a seizure how they can best help. If unable to prepare them ahead of time, be brief when you feel a warning sign as onset can occur rapidly. This will give you some control and it will help others to deal with the situation better and make sure that you are cared for.

The important thing for others to know is that you are not having an epileptic attack (there are no electrical discharge abnormalities occurring in your brain). Tell people ahead of time that they should avoid calling an ambulance unless you have injured yourself. Some people wear a medical bracelet that simply says "Non-epileptic seizures. No ambulance."

Also, you might carry a letter with you which would make others and an ambulance crew aware that your PNES are not epilepsy. This may stop them from giving you the wrong treatment.

These are my instructions to others on how to help when I am having a seizure:

Sit with me.

Protect my privacy as much as possible.
Speak to me calmly. I usually am able to hear and feel what people are doing when I have a seizure. Being spoken to in a calm reassuring manner can help to make my seizures shorter.

Put ice, if available, on the back of my neck. I have found that when I am having a seizure and more than one person is nearby, they feel like they need to do something to help. Applying ice to the back of the neck can be useful for some as the cold immediately eases the body when the sensation is directed to the neck area. It is only a palliative method of comfort for me and a form of comfort as well for my loved ones who want to be helpful during my seizures.

Keep me safe from injury. Help me to move if I am in an unsafe place. Or if that is not possible, move unsafe items away from me.

If I am on the floor, protect my head by carefully placing something soft under my head.

Do not try and restrict my movements.

Do not put anything in my mouth or try to give me medication.

Do not try to take my vital signs during a seizure. My seizures do not cause damage to my brain, even if they go on for several minutes.

Do not call an ambulance unless I am injured, completely unconscious, or having difficulty breathing. It is important that the ambulance crew know that my seizures are non-epileptic.

****

What do you want to tell people about how to care for you when you are having a seizure? Write it down here. Make copies for loved ones and others that might be with you during a seizure.

_____

_____

_____

_____

_____

_____

_____

_____

_____

_____

_____

_____

_____

After

We with PNES also experience a range of symptoms after our seizures. These may include tiredness and fatigue, changes in memory or speech, or changes in emotional state or physical sensations.

At the end of my seizures my right thigh muscles spasm and the pain is unbearable. I grab my leg and arch my back as my leg burns; it stiffens, and then it straightens out. My right arm and hand experience freezing cold sensations that last for about an hour. My neck is stiff and I have difficulty turning my head to the right. Often, I cannot remember what people have said during the event. I am very wobbly on my feet. If I can, I rest for a little while, but it usually takes around five hours for the exhaustion, nausea, and pain to wear off.

Other lasting side effects that I have experienced are short term memory issues, speech issues (aphasia) that causes me to say the wrong beginning of a word or an incorrect word that doesn't make sense in the sentence. Sometimes, I have issues with thinking. I also have balance issues. As days following the seizures lengthen into weeks, I find that the side effects soften. They had been very worrisome to me until I learned that many others with PNES have the same after effects.

What do I tell people?

Telling people that you have PNES can be difficult because, although many people have heard of epilepsy and know something about it, they have not heard of PNES.

PNES can be difficult to explain. Even telling others that the seizures from PNES do not include electrical discharge abnormalities within the brain, epilepsy does, may not help the cause of greater understanding.

Remember, if you have a good understanding of your diagnosis it will be easier to explain to others.

Here are some things you can say:

"I have been diagnosed with psychogenic non-epileptic seizures, also known as PNES."

"I have episodes that I cannot control. They are like epileptic seizures but they are not caused by the same things that cause epilepsy."

"Even though they are not epileptic, my seizures can still be very distressing for me."

"I have a condition similar to epilepsy, which means I have seizures."

****

How have you approached others to explain your seizures?

What did you say?

_____

_____

_____

_____

_____

_____

_____

_____

_____

_____

_____

_____

_____

_____

_____

_____

People may think that if you don't have epilepsy that your seizures are not real.

During a seizure in a management person's office, the person actually ordered me to cease the seizure! "Stop it! Stop it! Slap your leg! Make it stop! Slap your leg!" Of course, I couldn't. The person's response? "Get out of here! I can't stand looking at you!"

This shows others lack of knowledge about this condition.

Spread the word. The more people become aware, the less likely you will be treated in an undignified fashion.

We all use a range of coping strategies to help us deal with all the difficulties life throws at us. Different strategies are most effective for different situations. Like the proverbial 'elephant in the room', avoiding or pretending that problems don't exist can increase stress and cause problems to get bigger over time. An issue that one may not have resolved at an early point by talking about it or by asking someone to help may get so big that it causes the kind of stress which can start PNES.

All our concerns and emotions are very normal. Talking about them, learning to manage them, and getting our questions answered all form an important part of adapting and learning to cope with a diagnosis of PNES. Our treatment team can give us support.

And we look to loved ones who understand our diagnosis of non-epileptic seizures for support, encouragement, and yes, love.

Coping with your own feelings about your diagnosis can influence others' perceptions about non-epileptic seizures. Therefore, it can be helpful to explore your feelings and how they affect your behavior, the ways in which you act, and how you respond to yourself before, during, and after seizures.

I am fortunate to have my therapist and my psychiatrist as my team leaders for top notch support and encouragement.

Fast following are a very special person in my life, my family of loved ones, friends in the community and even people with whom I work who care about me. There are even some people who struggle with my diagnosis, I am sure, and who honor me as I am.

Consider talking about your feelings with family members, doctors, and others who have been diagnosed with PNES. There are web sites and pages on social sites like Facebook that will provide opportunities to talk through the written word as well.

Because PNES is a mind-body connected seizure disorder, it is crucial that we be able to seek help for our condition totally. Find a neurologist who is familiar with PNES. If you haven't yet, find a health care professional who has expertise in counseling and a psychiatrist who will be supportive and encouraging about PNES and prescribe medications as necessary for your care. Your primary care physician needs to be on board with your condition as well.

I had to provide some education and advocate for myself with my own physician.

Ask questions, get information. The more you understand about PNES and treatment options, the more this can help you gain some control of the situation.

Learning more about non-epileptic seizures can also help you to share appropriate information with others, as they too will most likely be trying to find ways to make sense of this diagnosis.

It is through advocating for ourselves and our own self-care that we find strength in ourselves. It is through connecting with others and sharing our experiences that we find that we are not alone.

It is when we accept our diagnosis of PNES and we accept ourselves as we are that we begin the emotional healing process.

What a blessing!

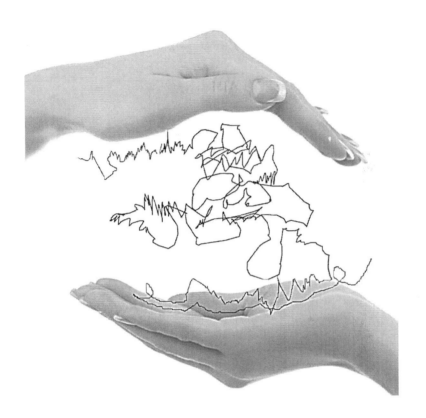

Embracing My Seizures

****

Scribble what your seizure looks like. Draw your hands too. Where are they in relation to the seizure scribble?

Are you able to encircle the seizure with your hands and embrace it?

Chapter 5 Opportunity For Grieving

There's a certain feeling of relief when an illness is given a name. I was searching and searching for answers while seizure after seizure occurred. PNES was my relief. Finally, what was happening to me had a name other than "pseudo-seizures" and "crying out for help," words that made me cringe.

However, while giving the seizures the name PNES helped me immensely, my reaction to every seizure then and every seizure since... I HATE THEM!

I hate the shaking. I hate the jerking, bending, and twisting. I hate the crying. I hate the swearing. I hate the burning pain and spasms.

I hate knowing that there will be another seizure, then another, and still another seizure. I hate knowing that one more seizure, one more bang up seizure will end the cluster. I hate not knowing the time that it will occur.

Even more, I hate having seizures in public. Never mind the seizure of which I have no control. It's being hypersensitive and conscious during my seizures that causes me embarrassment, guilt, and shame that I feel especially with strangers.

I hate the after effects: memory loss, aphasia, and poor balance. They are my perception and reminders of what I've lost.

It's what I've lost that provides me with the positive opportunity to grieve. You may wonder how grieving can be positive.

I don't know anyone personally who has PNES. However, the communication I build with others through my contact via websites such as **http://nonepilepticseizures.com** and social media, I feel like I know many persons who have and are now processing the grief that comes from experiencing these non-epileptic seizures. We are sharing it all together. Surely, none of us has asked for them to occur. Surely, none of us enjoys the experience of having seizures. While I am not totally debilitated from my seizures, they affect my physical health, my mental wellbeing, and my spirit as well. I have felt many emotions that are connected directly with grief.

Grief is emotional suffering felt when something or someone loved is taken away. The more significant the loss, the more intense the grief will be. Grief may be associated with the death of a loved one which is often the cause of the most intense type of grief. In addition, even a subtle loss can cause grief, including the loss of health.

Everyone grieves differently; experiencing and working through the grief process is very individual and personal for each of us. How we grieve depends on many factors, including our personality and coping style, our life experience, our faith, and the nature of the loss. The grieving process takes time. Healing happens gradually. It can neither be forced nor hurried, nor is there a set timetable for grieving. Whatever our grief experience, it's important to be patient with ourselves and allow the process to naturally unfold.

Consider when "psychogenic non-epileptic seizures" or "PNES" was first spoken to you in a diagnosis. Having gained the knowledge that you are now challenged with this condition, you may have experienced the following:

Shock and disbelief –

It may have been easier to have heard the word epilepsy - a neurological disorder marked by sudden recurrent episodes of sensory disturbance, loss of consciousness, or convulsions, associated with abnormal electrical activity in the brain, than to hear that the seizures are non-epileptic and occur as a result of combined psychological experiences impacting the body; that these seizures highly involve issues of mental health. I know that I didn't want to hear that I am faced with yet another mental health concern.

Anger –

The seizures are not anyone's fault. Those affected can't control when they happen. Having the non-epileptic seizures made me incredibly angry. I was and still feel anger towards myself for having them. I blamed and still blame myself for having them. I asked my Higher Power, why, what else, and why again. I still wait for answers.

Guilt –

Feeling guilty about knowing that the seizures come from the mind and that what happened to us developmentally has caused the seizures to surface can affect us. We may think that if we had done something differently in our lives the deep mental anguish would not occur. We may feel guilty having to explain that the seizures are non-epileptic, yet they are a serious condition. I think that guilt and shame go hand in hand. I have experienced guilt and shame too when I am out of control as to when, where, and why the seizures happen and I feel the need to tell others what is going on, almost to justify the seizures in my defense of them and my defense of me. That is guilt and shame at work. I also often feel guilty and ashamed when I know that my seizures stem from traumatic occurrences that have happened to me even as I may not precisely remember what the agonizing emotional disturbances were.

Fear –

Having PNES can for some trigger a host of worries and fears. People with this challenge may feel helpless, anxious, and insecure. Some may even have panic attacks. For me, I worry when the next seizure will occur. I worry where it will occur. The seizures at times make me anxious, especially if they occur at work. I worry that my job will be affected. My job was significantly affected several years ago. My spirit worries because of my perception that with yet another medical-mental health condition, I won't be acceptable to my loved ones. I worry that I might be loved less. I realize that this fear is my own perception, but it affects me much.

Sadness –

This is probably the most universal emotion of grief. We may experience feelings of emptiness, despair, or deep loneliness. We may cry a lot and feel mentally and emotionally unstable. My lack of hope, my feeling of isolation, and the sensations of emptiness have lessened over time, but I admit that crying a lot and feeling mentally and emotionally unstable following a bout of seizures happens to me quite often.

There are physical symptoms that accompany grief often times. Fatigue, nausea, lowered immunity, weight loss or weight gain, aches and pains, and insomnia as well; not to mention our individual side effects from the seizures themselves can be felt along with the emotional reactions. It never occurred to me that all the signs and symptoms that I had were a physical response to grief.

Finding the support of other persons is the most important thing that we can do for ourselves as we experience and work through our grief. Even if we take pride in being strong and self-sufficient, there will be times to lean on others who can support and encourage us. Psychiatrist and/or therapist alike are trained to listen to us objectively. When grief feels as if it's too much to bear, a mental health professional with experience in grief counseling will help us work through intense emotions and overcome obstacles to our grieving. They will assist us to find the ways that aid us in coping with our PNES. I am fortunate to find one hundred percent (and what feels like even more) support from my own therapist and psychiatrist.

Drawing loved ones close rather than avoiding them and accepting what they can offer is very paramount to our healing. We can confide in our trusted friends. I have a time honored friend and a special loved one who provides support for me no end. In their own way they encourage me and my loved one even nudges me when I need that.

Embracing a faith or spiritual practice can provide comfort. Spirit minded activities can offer solace.
Sharing our feelings about PNES with others who have

experienced or are experiencing grief alongside us can be a boon. If anyone is fortunate enough to find a face to face support group through a medical professional, how great that could be!

Reading about our condition and sharing with others can often provide comfort for us.

We especially need to look after our physical health. The mind and body are glued together and closely connected with our non-epileptic seizures. When we feel better physically, we will feel better emotionally. It's important for us to get enough sleep, eat right, engage in some form of exercise and fill our spirits with pleasurable activities too.

We cannot allow anyone to tell us how to feel and we shouldn't command ourselves how to feel either. Our grief is our own; no one else, including ourselves, can tell us when it's time to move on or to get over it. We need to let grief happen as it does in its own time. We need to let ourselves feel whatever we feel without embarrassment or judgment. It's okay to be angry, to yell at the heavens, to cry or not to cry. It's also okay to laugh, to find moments of joy, and to let go when we're ready and we find acceptance within.

My only caveat here is that if the level of grief freezes at a particular level, remains intrusively significant over a lengthy period of time, it may be a moment to consider getting professional support.

****

Since hearing that you have PNES, have you experienced grief? Are you experiencing grief at this time? Did you wonder then or do you wonder now what your feelings have been all about? Give yourself permission to feel that grief.

Release and organize your feelings by writing them out.
You will feel better for it.

_____
_____
_____
_____
_____
_____
_____
_____
_____
_____
_____
_____
_____
_____
_____
_____
_____
_____
_____
_____
_____
_____
_____
_____

Chapter 6 So Much More

Never forget. We are not defined by our PNES! We are persons who are challenged with this mind-body condition.

That's all.

We are defined by so much more!

Admittedly, when I was in the throes of seizure after seizure with no diagnosis and nowhere to get any answers or assistance physically and mentally, I was one-hundred percent focused on my seizures. I was stuck in the frightening unknown. I forgot about all the good things that define me. I forgot that I have so many gifts inside me. I forgot that there are so many opportunities for me.

Now, when I have the seizures, I do feel horrible. I go through all my emotions. I even grieve again for a few minutes. But then I acknowledge the seizures and accept them for what they are: minutes of agony. While I hate the seizures and hours of after effects, the days and weeks of side effects, I don't live those feelings twenty four hours a day, seven days a week. Why should I dwell on them and the negative feelings and emotions when I have so many other positive aspects to myself and so many things that I need to do and want to do?

The feeling of loss is done. The joy of life is back and we are ready for it!

We have PNES, yes. We have so many possibilities beyond too.

I know it feels so much easier to write the negative things about us. However, we have so much more that is good and positive.

Take some time now to write down your positive attributes. After that, add some of the possibilities in your life, remembering that you are not your seizures. You are exceptional and unusual. You are remarkably unique. You are a marvel.

Dig a little if you have to. (Shhh...I had to dig for a while too).

_____
_____
_____
_____
_____
_____
_____
_____
_____
_____
_____
_____
_____
_____
_____
_____
_____
_____
_____
_____
_____
_____
_____
_____
_____

In my chosen career, I work primarily with elders in a healthcare setting. The focus of my work is to help the elders bring meaning, purpose, joy, and peace into their lives. I am required to provide activities in the areas of five basic needs: physical, emotional, mental, social, and spiritual.

Many of the elders suffer from depression, anxiety, and loneliness derived from the grief they work through as they deal with many losses of their own. To observe smiles and see other signs of pleasure is a joy to me, knowing that they are feeling better at least for that moment in the day. I am pleased when I create many moments of sweet emotions.

Sometimes, due to the effects of our PNES, many of us find ourselves becoming introverted, spending much time alone.

It isn't good to spend day after day alone. We need interaction with others for balanced mental health. Spending too much time alone can even affect our brain function.

Applying the five basic needs into our own activities of our daily lives may ease how we feel about and deal with our PNES as we find meaning, purpose, joy, and peace within ourselves.

Taking care of our physical, emotional, mental, social, and spiritual selves will bring wellness to our minds, hearts, and spirits.

PNES is more easily managed if our lives are balanced through activities that provide us with a steady positive journey through our days. It is okay to cry, but it is also beneficial to smile and even laugh. Many of us forget that. The components of the five basic needs are all integrated and influence one another.

Here are some suggestions for each category. Each of us finds what makes us feel best.

Physical -

Find a doctor who supports you and encourages you and

honors the PNES and treats you well. Keep up with physical exams and tests as needed and ordered.

Find a therapist and psychiatrist who treat PNES. You will most likely take some medication. You will both need and want to share. You want someone who listens and offers encouragement.

The stress alone of having PNES can bring on all kinds of physical complaints and illnesses. Moving the body, especially through exercise can increase endorphins, the feel good hormones.

Find some exercise that will be pleasurable: walking, exercise class, yoga, tai chi, even dance.

Go for a hike; bring a friend along.

Go to sleep and awaken at the same time daily through the week and get enough rest. Sleep 8 hours or whatever your body requires. A daily short nap is refreshing too.

Eat three meals a day and drink enough water.

Acute Stress + Anxiety + Exhaustion = Seizures for me. It is imperative that I strive to get enough sleep and release tension through exercise. I found a dance exercise program that is perfect for me. I even look forward to the hours of exercise!

Emotional-

Happiness comes from within. Learning to meet our own emotional needs will help us cope with our seizures.

Recognize when your emotions affect your body.

Express your needs and feelings.

Express your opinions appropriately.

Smile!

Laugh! Use humor to lighten the negative thoughts.

Cry when you need to; crying helps release tension.

Sit by yourself for a few minutes in quiet. Notice your thoughts as they arise. Get to know your mind.

Use journal writing to express your thoughts; that will help relieve your stress.

Talk to a trusted friend. Talk to your loved ones.

Find ways to be grateful.

Find ways to give to yourself and to others.

When you're afraid, anxious, insecure or totally overwhelmed, make an appointment with your therapist/psychiatrist.

Find ways to release anger. Beat a pillow.

Years ago, a therapist told me to take a rock and give it the identity of my anger and then throw it. I did that physically for a long time. Now, I can say out loud, "I need to throw rocks!"

Share touch. Give and receive lots of hugs.

Believe in yourself and your abilities. Be optimistic.

Mental/Intellectual and Social go hand in hand-

It's good for your brain when you challenge yourself.

Learn something new.

Read. Read. Read.
Write in your journal.

Try this with your opposite hand: brush your teeth, comb

your hair, fasten buttons, eat, and write. This kind of work actually gives your brain a workout.

Take advantage of new experiences and opportunities both by yourself and with friends and loved ones.

Develop relationships where both you and the other person feel good.

Share lively conversations.

Choose a goal and reward yourself when you have accomplished it.

Find support for PNES where you can share your experience and your feelings.

Deep breathing can help the mind body connection and ease tense emotions.

Spiritual -

Nourish your spirit through personal beliefs, morals, and/or practicing faith or religion.

Develop a philosophy of life that you want to live by.

Feel connected with yourself and others.

Identify your emotions. Express your emotions.

Have a place where you can relax; chill out.

After work, make a purposeful transition from work to home. Change your clothes, take a shower, etc.

Find purpose in your life and meaning in all of the things you do in a day.

Give your sense of taste a treat. Experience the flavor of something that for you is divine.

Take a yoga class.

Find music that soothes and brings joy.

Read and write affirmations.

Meditate.

Jot down some ideas that will give you the opportunity to really experience your mind-body connection.

_____

_____

_____

_____

_____

_____

_____

_____

_____

_____

_____

_____

_____

_____

_____

_____

_____

_____

_____

_____

Chapter 7 Holistic Self-care

Being healthy encompasses all our parts, not just our physical body. When our emotions are in turmoil or our mind is bombarded with obsessive thoughts our health is compromised and we already know the result equals seizures. It is important to create balance in our lives by nurturing our entire selves. It is paramount to our total health to meet our spiritual, mental, emotional, and physical needs.

This nurturing should be holistic, taking into consideration who we are and how we feel totally. When we care for ourselves holistically, we give attention to our mind, our body, and our spirit.

The body, mind and spirit work as one. They join to keep vitality and life flowing within us. Depending on our state of being in every moment, our feeling of vigor and sparkle can change constantly.

Our state of being is our overall feeling of health, wellness, and how balanced we feel on all levels of our being. Whether we are happy or sad, sick or well, connected to our spirit or not, we are either in or out of balance with whom we really are.

If we feel balanced, we will experience joy in what we do. We will have a sense of purpose and feel that our lives have meaning. We will treat ourselves with love and respect. We will also be loving and respectful with our loved ones. We will feel calm and less stressed and anxious. That can lead to a quieting of our seizures.

It's plain to see that when we are not balanced we will experience the exact opposite of what is positive in our lives. Our goal then should be to seek that balance. We should find harmony and peace within ourselves first and then seek peace and harmony with our loved ones and the world around us.

There is a natural flow from our body, mind, and spirit that creates our own balanced energy. If negative in nature, that flow creates our seizures! What we do in any given moment affects our life balance completely.

Life alone, never mind our seizures, can get in the way of being balanced. Taking care of ourselves as best we can with the support of as-needed professionals, along with our loved ones who will love, care about, and support us is our opportunity for the balance that we seek.

The activities and the reflective questions on the following pages will provide an opportunity for you to enjoy a body, mind, and spirit experience. They are shown first to give you examples of what you'll find in the itinerary of the three day retreat that follows in the next chapter.

The activities are simple, inexpensive, and fun ways to make a connection with you.

The reflective questions are opportunities to examine and express your emotions and feelings.

The Personal Three Day Retreat that follows is a guide to give you quiet self-care. It is designed to be uniquely your own experience. The guide is only that - you will find suggestions and opportunities for your own choices towards wellness.

Be blessed with healing in your body, mind, and spirit. May your seizures be quieted.

Experience Color

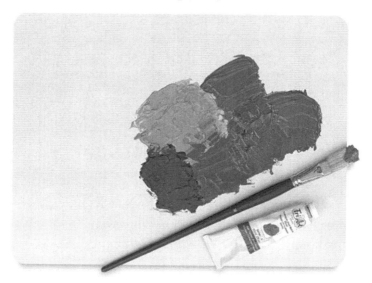

Experience Color (by painting)

What color represents your seizures? Immerse yourself in the color. It's amazing the feelings that putting the color down on paper can stir.

Materials:

Watercolor paint.

Brush(es).

Paper - watercolor paper is best if possible, but sketch paper or any plain paper will do.

Medium size cup of water.

Once you decide on the color, brush it onto the paper. Use more water to make the paint a thin wash or less water to produce a more intense color. Be free with the brush; let it decide how to move and put down the color

Color a Mandala

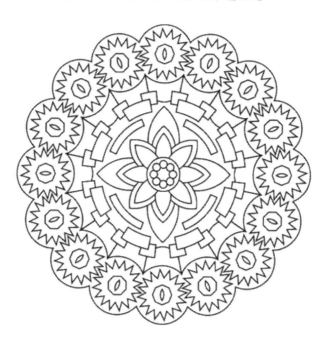

Color a Mandala

There are books available for purchase and even patterns to print for free online. Coloring can be a peaceful distraction helping us to focus our attention in a repetitive pattern. It's soothing.

Materials:

Mandala patterned drawing.

Colored pencils, crayons, markers.

Whatever color you choose, repeat that color in the same pattern around the mandala. No need to rush. Take all the time you need to complete.

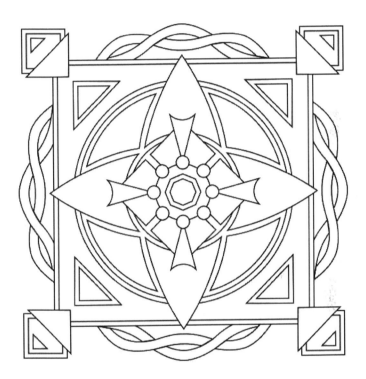

Pleasant emotions emerge with modeling clay play :)

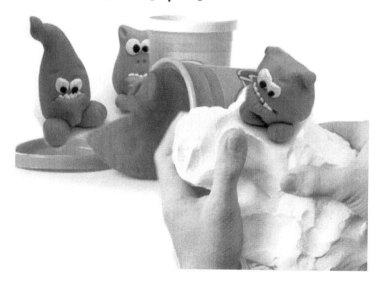

Modeling Clay Play

Nothing says stress relief like squeezing, squishing, rolling, and even pounding clay to get the emotions out. Modeling clay...it's not just for kids.

Materials:

Modeling clay or Play-doh - try different colors. Surface to work on, follow directions on clay if paper needs to be used.

Dig right in. Hold the clay; warm it in your hands. What emotions are you feeling? Take it out on the clay. Feel a sense of humor? Show it through what you form out of the clay.

Homemade playing dough

1 cup flour
1 cup water
1/3 cup salt
2 teaspoons cream of tartar
1 tablespoon vegetable oil

Mix all ingredients together in a medium size pan. Cook over medium temperature. Stir constantly. Mixture will thicken, appear lumpy, and then pull away from the sides of the pan. Instant dough! Turn out onto flat surface. Let cool for a couple minutes then knead. It's ready for squishing, rolling, modeling, and stress relieving. It's great to work with it while it's warm :)

Music...
the universal language of
mind, heart, and spirit

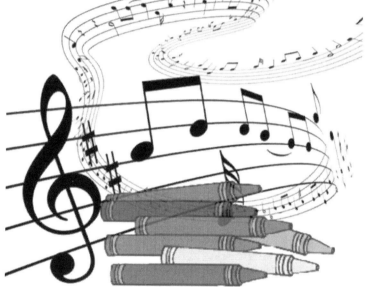

Music, Universal Language of Mind and Heart

Drawing or coloring to music will touch your senses. The combination will have unique revelations for you.

Materials:

Choose a selection of music that you really like.

Paper.

Crayons, colored markers, watercolors, colored pencils, etc.

As the music begins, close your eyes and hear the notes; see the colors. Let your mind wander as you let the colors wander. Expect a feeling of peace to wash over you.

Black Out Poetry

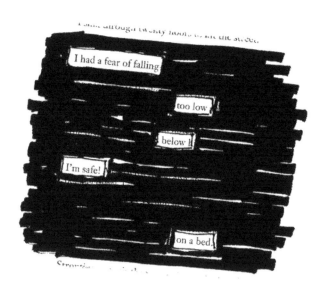

Black Out Poetry

It's amazing when reading through an article or a page of a book how words can pop out at you and help you say what you want to say.

Materials needed:

Newspaper article or a page from an old book.

Fine black marker.

Sharpie or thicker marker.

Directions - Look through the article or page of a book. Find random words that would go together to express your thoughts. With the fine marker draw a rectangle around the word. Leave a little more space even going into letters nearby as the marker will bleed slightly. Fill in and cover all the rest of the words, leaving your thought, your poem.

Torn Paper
Collage

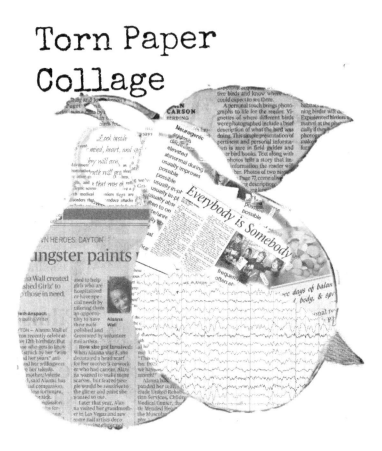

Torn Paper Collage

Within the collage, I like to use phrases, words, or pictures that convey my thoughts and feelings.

Materials:

Glue stick or white glue, Elmer's type.

Sheet of paper with a simple picture on it. Magazines, newspapers, anything to tear and form the collage.

Find a picture or draw one. Tear pieces of magazine pages, matching colors of the picture underneath or use newspaper in torn pieces. Glue the torn pieces to the picture.

COLOR YOUR SEIZURES

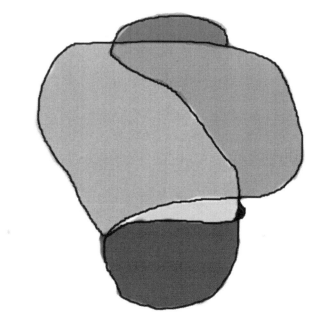

Color Your Seizures

What do your seizures look like? Release the seizure
in a free drawing on paper, then color each section
to represent how the seizures look and feel.

Materials:

Paper.

Pen, pencil, or fine point marker.

*Crayons, colored markers, watercolors, colored
pencils, etc.*

Put the pen to paper and begin drawing your seizure
squiggle. Let the pen take your hand where it will.
Close the squiggle and color in each section. You will
reveal your colors inside as well.

Affirmation Mandala

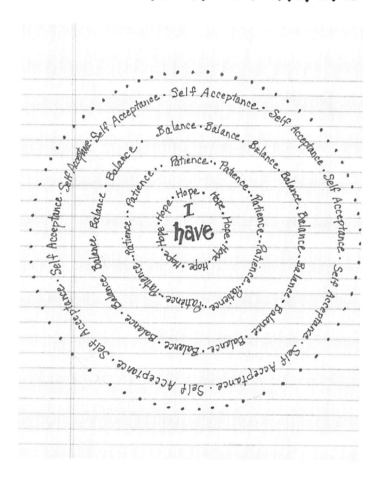

Affirmation Mandala

Remember when you were in school and the teacher had a student write on the chalkboard over and over a sentence or a phrase so that it was ingrained in their mind and they would never forget it? An affirmation mandala is similar, but in a very positive way. Affirmations are written over and over until the pleasant sayings sink into your spirit.

Materials:

Paper.

Pen or pencil.

A plate or circular object to trace onto the paper.

Trace the largest circle on the paper. Smaller circles can be drawn free hand within the larger circle or other circular items can be used to trace. There should be four circles for the affirmations leading into the center of the smallest circle.
In the center, focus on yourself. Write "I ___" I chose the words "I have.." What are the affirmations that you want to say to yourself? Write each word or phrase over and over around the circles. Decorate the edge and in between the words if you desire. Keep the affirmations close at hand in your mind and heart.

Reflections of self...

Look inside

your mind, heart, and spirit

They will awaken &

your truth will grace the pen

Peace that was one hidden

will begin to surface

Kate Taylor

Reflective Questions

1. What are the things that stand between you and complete happiness?

2. How would you describe yourself in 5 words?

3. What would you do differently if you knew that no one was judging you?

4. If you could ask a single person one question, and they must answer honestly what would you ask?

5. Are you holding onto something that you need to let go of?

6. How do you celebrate the things you do have in your life?

7. If you had a friend that you spoke to the same way you speak to yourself, how long do you think that person would allow you to be your friend?

8. If you had to teach someone one thing, what would you teach?

9. What makes you smile?

10. What can you do today that you couldn't do a year ago? What will you be able to do at this time next year?

11. What do you want most out of life?

12. If you could go back in time, once, and change a single thing, what would it be?

13. If you could ask for one wish, what would it be?

14. What did you want to be when you were a kid?

15. What terrifies you the most?

16. What are you looking forward to?

17. Describe the greatest adventure of your life.

18. What have you done that you're most proud of?

19. What is your greatest strength?

20. What is your greatest weakness?

21. What bad habits do you want to break?

22. Would you rather have 10 years of excellent health, or 30 years of average health?

23. How much control do you really have over yourself?

24. If you could only keep five possessions, what would they be?

25. What teacher in school made the most impact on you?

26. If you won the lottery, what would you do?

27. What are your top three favorite books and why?

28. What are you most afraid of?

29. What was your most embarrassing moment?

30. What age do you feel right now and why?

31. How would your friends describe you?

32. Do you think crying is a sign of weakness or strength?

33. What lifts your spirits when life gets you down?

34. What are your favorite simple pleasures?

35. You are not alone having PNES. How does that feel?

The Most Delicious Pear I Have Ever Tasted

I have written it down
Told the story more times than my fingers can count
Recalled with fondness
The memory
Of the deliciousness of you.
The first year
Not knowing what to expect
I remember moving from one experience to the other
Just trying to follow the order of things.
Ahh, but the second year
I knew what to do
So I could relax
And let myself take it all in.
The experience of
Silent Retreat
Not far from home, really
But seemingly, so far away
Another world...
Of quiet
Save for the thirty minutes daily
That we could visit with one another.
Our time was spent listening
Listening to lectures
Listening to scriptures
Listening to music
Listening to nature
And the very sound of our breathing
For a couple days...
Reveling in the sound of silence
Shhh...
The very quietness itself
Awakened my senses
The sounds in my mind as I thought
About the readings,
Listening to what He was saying to me.
To ME!
But I remember so vividly
The taste of the food
Prepared by the Carmelites

Soup... vegetable, rich broth, so simple
Yet a symphony of flavors and textures
Bread... warm, earthy, speckled with seeds
Nurturing, sopping up the broth so as
To not miss a drop.
Water...clear, no hint of bleach or chemicals
Flavorless? Maybe flavor filled with taste of life.
But it was the pear
The single succulent pear
Whose taste I best recall!
Fat, green and freckled
Not perfect by any means
The skin wielding to the touch
Of my fingertip
Oh so ready
For that first bite,
Juice trickles down my chin.
The graininess of the flesh sticks to my teeth
The fragrance, so fresh, permeates my nostrils
And the memory of that taste
Is pleasantly burned into my mind.
Focusing with all my senses
On that one piece of fruit
Taking my time to enjoy the pleasure of each taste
Touch, smell, look,
Listening to the sound of mmmm
The totally sensual delight
I had never tasted deliciousness like that
In a simple pear.
Nor will I ever again.
What a gift!

Kate Taylor

Chapter 8 Embracing and Blending

For the want to recreate the taste of that perfect pear, I created my personal three day retreat. For the want of a pear! My lips, my mind, and my spirit craved it!

With the stress of daily life surrounding me, I welcomed my yearly retreat at the Carmelite monastery in a nearby town. The weekend was so quiet and peace filled. Each year I enjoyed the silence and gentleness of the three days that I left the world behind. When I returned to my world and back to the crazy busy life I kept a peace within for at least a little while.

The monastery burned down in a tragic fire. The Carmelites left.

I was depressed and alone inside. I wanted that peace again.

I couldn't travel, so I decided to create my own weekend of solitude and solace.

I kept the itinerary of my own retreat very much the same as the retreats at the monastery. Meals at the guided retreats were very simple: freshly baked bread, light flavorful soups, garden-fresh vegetables, cheeses and fruit. One glass of homemade wine each day, and oh, yes...the pear. Every year I had to include one pear. I sought the taste of the first, but alas it still has never returned to me.

I set aside three days of vacation time just for myself. Wednesday through Friday were the days that worked best for me and would lead me into a restful weekend.
I planned my daily itinerary and prepared for my creative time in advance. I purchased a journal that was pleasing to my eyes; I would keep it only for my retreat.

My daily mindful walk would be spirit led. My Higher Power would show me where to walk and what to see. One day, I noticed so many old stone walls. When I wrote in my journal about my walk, the symbolism of stone walls as boundaries came to my mind. That was significant for me.

Another day on my mindful walk I was led to go to a spot that had been a sad depressing place for me. I was able to walk the little street and stop at the place. I closed my eyes. I was shaking and my breaths came too shallow, but I stood where I needed to. I opened my eyes. I was okay. I turned and looked. The sun shone down on the place and I was okay. I walked away feeling lighter and hopeful, so happy that I had achieved overcoming that sadness.

Reading filled me with solace. I picked a tranquil book.

The creative activities made me smile. They felt a little silly at first, but my heart warmed as my hands were busy. Meditation and quiet time let me drift away. The quiet was comfort wrapped around me.

The most difficult part when I began the retreat was not turning off the TV; it was shutting down the computer and then phone. My lifelines!! Admittedly, I did go thru some withdrawal for a little time the first day, but I survived and welcomed the time alone with no distractions.

The guide for Embracing & Blending" The Color of Seizures Retreat" is yours to personalize.

I have outlined an itinerary for you. I recommend making the retreat for three days, but make the time away from the busy-ness of your own life your own. If you desire only one day, even just part of a day for your time of quiet and solace, by all means do what is comfortable for you.

With all your senses, experience this time for yourself. See everything with new eyes. Breathe in the aromas that come to you. Taste the deliciousness of your own 'pear'. Listen to the Spirit who speaks within you. And touch with new sensations in your fingertips.

Give yourself the gift of the retreat. You are precious and deserve this time. It will provide you with peace which in turn will soften your anxiety and stress. When you feel lighter your seizures will soften too.

Many blessings on your retreat.

My prayer for you is to find support, hope, love, and peace with your PNES.

Know that you are cared about and loved. You are not alone.

Note: This retreat is a quiet one. No television, No computer Give your mind the rest it deserves.

Embracing & Blending the Color of Seizures

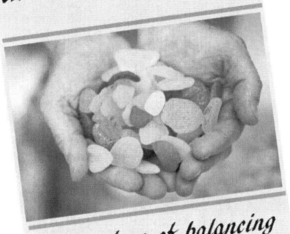

Three days of balancing mind, body, & spirit

Annual personal retreat for those with PNES

Psychogenic Non-epileptic Seizures

Embracing and Blending the Color of Seizures
Three days of balancing mind, body, and spirit.

8:00 - 8:30   Spirit Time - However you practice your spiritual beliefs.

8:30 - 9:00   Breakfast - Natural cereal, yogurt, fruit, juice, coffee or tea.

9:30 - 10:00   Reading - Select something gentle and inspiring.

10:00 - 11:00   Mindful Walk - Go where your Spirit leads you. Let your mind be open to experience what will be a treasure for you.

11:00 - 12:00   Journaling about the walk.

12:00 - 1:00   Lunch and free time - Soup, salad, bread, butter, fruit, and one small glass of wine if desired.

1:30 - 2:30   Meditation Rest - Close your eyes and be open to your spirit's gifts. If you find yourself drifting into a gentle sleep, let it happen.

2:30 - 3:00   Creative Activity - Choose something from the list or immerse yourself in the form of art you desire.

3:00 - 4:00   Reflective Questions – choose one or more from the list. Give yourself plenty of time to collect your thoughts and write about the questions in your journal.

You are not alone, and you are not controlled by PNES.

Feel the balance that you are achieving. Feel how your body, mind, and spirit are becoming one.
Feel the peace that comes to you. It's a blessing!

The poems included in this book are my journey through the pain of not knowing about what was happening to me. Writing kept my body, mind, and spirit connected. I look back at them now and see the excruciating pain, but I no longer relive it. I now know PNES is part of me and I accept it. My journey to healing continues.

MRI

Until I release it,
My mind cleaves to such memories as this:
Bound, braced and locked into my own coffin
Made comfortable all the same
For what would seem like an eternity
In daylight darkness.
Caretaker said the last good-bye
And closed the cover.
Opened eyes.
Closed eyes.
Breathed.
Why bother? There seemed no way out
Tongue adhered to the roof of my mouth
Instructed this way "Do NOT swallow."
The pianist played music for me
Did anyone sing?
Did anyone stand to pray?
The thunderous noise
Pounding!
Crashing down!
Crashing in!
And then
I was being dismembered

Flesh slashed away from bone
Readied for a sky burial
Angel winged vultures
Each took a morsel
Of me
Carried me away.
And after a taste
Discarded the shard of my bone
Over highlands, sea
And barren desert
To my rest then?
No.
It was neither time then, nor time now
For departure.
Instead
I arose and returned
Bones cut and scarred
Ready to hear
The answer to the question.

Personal Earthquake

All I wanted was a drink of water.

I opened the fridge door

Cool air and condiments lit with a glow.

I saw the bottle; it was right there.

Suddenly sensing seismic activity,

I was an earthquake!

Heavy door cut into the pit of my left arm.

I could not free myself from that white behemoth!

As I trembled and shook from head to toe,

The door quivered, the entire refrigerator rocked!

The earthquake that was me

Jiggled the bowls on top of the fridge!

I couldn't free myself from the refrigerator door

Or from the shaking, bending, pounding of my own body

Or the twisting, swearing, crying!

I was seizing!

The bowls rattled forward, taking steps toward the edge.

I was conscious through it all and conscious that the

Blue sponge painted heavy popcorn bowl,

Grammy's white antique mixing bowl,

My favorite Pyrex bowl and that

Little vintage one, just the right size,

Could easily fall on me and crash into mosaic pieces

With me underneath them

If the seizure didn't stop soon!

Why the hell was I worried about the precious bowls?!

The entire refrigerator could have collapsed on top of me!

In what felt like more than a couple minutes,

My earthquake, at least a five on the Richter scale, ceased.

The only seizure I had ever experienced completely

While standing left me physically and emotionally weak.

Released and wobbly, I sat on the floor.

So thirsty.

Kate Taylor

White Flag

No more quips.
No more quotes,
No more cutesy pie.
Today, I am in pain.
Today, I am powerless.
You said you want it.
You said you'd take it.
Well, you can have it.
All of it.
I hand it over.
You fix it.
Amen

Desert Journey

I don't remember how long I had trudged alone
Through this desert
Lips parched
Cheeks burned from sun and windblown sand
Eyes squinting and irritated.
At night I froze in place as the sun went down.
Nothing ahead of me.
Oh, I had experienced the mirage of oasis
Palm trees and cleansing refreshing water
But as I reached out to take it,
It slipped through my hands
Like the sand that sifted between my finger.
I met more than a precious few along my journey
Who offered solace and sustenance?

Guidance for direction?
But the passage was still my own.
I lay prostrate in the dust
Exhausted and fearful
Afraid that I would never rise again,
Sand sweeping over me.
Not a grain of it successful.
The jerking of my limbs
Kept me from being buried
Until you took my hand in yours
Lifted me
Offered me the tiniest crumb
And a sip of water.
Another mirage?
Not this time.

This oasis was to become my place of respite.
Palm trees, luscious fruit and drink
Billowing sheer voile
Gentle breeze
The softest place to cradle my head
Flannel or 600 count Egyptian cotton
It mattered not then, not now.
Before long
I found the slumber
that I had long searched for

Rest at last.

Spoken Words

The air was steamy
As sea salty droplets
Washed over her as healing took place.

Earlier that day,
She saw his eyes.
He spoke her name
And then with head lowered,
He began to pour through her life's story.

She hesitated for a moment
And chose to speak
Before the fear once again took over.

She said, "Please, before we go any further,
I need your full attention. Look at me now."

Who knew that taking him with her to
Experience her pain, and embrace her feelings
Would be paramount to her healing?

He stopped.
He listened.
She spoke.

With pen in hand, words were written
That affected her life in a daunting way.
Those very words tainted others' perception of her,
And she became stigmatized.

He had to hear and know this.

She spoke.

He listened.
He heard.
And then he knew.

He asked, "Do I need to apologize?"

She responded, "No. Not anymore."

What she needed was for him to be aware.
Aware that some words written
Appear as God spoken.

She spoke. She really spoke!
The words she spoke that day
Were God given, God spoken.

She was empowered.

He spoke. "You have courage. And, I am sorry."
She smiled.

They embraced.
She was able to let go
Emotionally, spiritually and physically.

The healing began.

Kate Taylor

About the Authors

Kate Taylor is nationally certified as an Activities Director and has award winning history working in Activities in long term care and is a Licensed Nursing Assistant as well. She is a poet; also talented in the world of watercolor and enjoys playing the piano.

Some say that no one lives in New Hampshire, but Kate does. She resides in the small town of Jaffrey and she has much to share in the way of writing.

Her first work as an established author is entitled, "The Pink Eraser."

Jeffrey Underwood graduated from the University of Washington with a degree in psychology, though he has practiced as a Registered Nurse for many years. He also comes from a family of traditionally published authors. His first published work was the "Forbidden Tome; Hansel and Gretel's True Tale." His second was entitled "Lethal Assumed; Lost Tome Found." Three more books followed in the Entity Saga and now, eleven in Sarah's Saga. Sarah's Saga, written dually, fall under his and coauthor Kate Taylor's rubric.

He currently resides in Mountlake Terrace, Washington, a suburb of Seattle and hopes that those who read the just published, "Sting of the Golden Bee," part of Sarah's Saga, also co-written with Kate Taylor, will become aware of yet another slice of significant human history as the new tale speaks about the early origins of the country of France and how that nation was formed out of a barbaric and tidal dynasty known as the Merovingians. They are currently working on the next tale in Sarah's Saga, "Sea Of Impulse."

Kate has collaborated with Jeff on many a novel now. The earliest of their collaborations were entitled "Treason's Truth; Mac Alpin's Scotland," "Eagle's Eclipse; America Before Columbus," "Tasman's Travail; The Journey Down Under," and "Highland Gals."

Their more recent tales have been "Sonnet In Red Ink," "Tracks of Lost Tears," and "Captive To Cocoa." The sad fact of child slavery in the chocolate industry is revealed in the final of those three. The entire compilation of Sarah's Saga includes:" Eyes of A Pagan Queen," "White Scream," "Scythian Sorrows," "Indecent Diane," "Glitter's Graveyard," "Crist Miss Blues," "Skin Monster," "Sunset Over The Villerouge," "Honor's Implacable Soldier," and their newest, "Sting of the Golden Bee." It now will include the soon to be published "Sea Of Impulse."

Both Kate and Jeff hope that" The Color Of Seizures" brings a sense of balance and peace to those who, like Kate, are challenged with PNES.

Kate and Jeff are presently immersed in developing their own publishing and consulting business.

On a playful level, Kate and Jeff have also combined in writing "The Rule of Thumb & Fingers," a texter's bible with lots of laughs, and "Sock Monkey Life," which is full of sheer creativity.

Jeff and Kate met online and found that their collaborative interests meshed splendidly. This new novel is an example of that blending of gusto for writing that they both certainly have.

"Many authors write only a few books in a lifetime. Kate and I have written nearly a dozen in a year. You might ask, does quantity sacrifice quality here? It doesn't happen to. That's why this occurrence is so exceptional. Kate and I love our characters. There is a reason for that. It's because it is truly a captivating world. Writing is a love affair. Until you have found it, you will never know the potential depth of it. Kate and I have found it." - Jeff Underwood

By the by, despite a distance of three thousand miles, for nearly four years now, Kate and Jeff have accomplished the writing and self-publishing of their books via texts, email, or phone alone. They have yet to meet. But they will.

Books by Jeffrey Underwood & Kate Taylor

TREASONS TRUTH-BAD ASS HAPPENINGS OCCURING IN EARLY SCOTLAND.

EAGLE'S ECLIPSE-THE MYSTERIOUS DISAPPEARANCE OF A THRIVING AMERICAN INDIAN CITY.

TASMAN'S TRAVAIL-THE DISTURBING IMPACT OF EUROPEAN COLONIZATION OF NEW ZEALAND.

EYES OF A PAGAN QUEEN-A WOMAN'S JOURNEY INTO EARLY ETHIOPEAN TREATMENT OF A CHRISTIAN EMPIRE.

WHITE SCREAM-A SCREAMING PLEA PRESENT DAY NONVIOLENCE AND COOPERATION.

SCYTHIAN SORROWS-A MOURNING MOTHER'S PATH TO HER ONCE DECEASED SON.

HIGHLAND GALS-THE JOURNEY IN NURTURING IN THE LIFE OF FOUR MIDDLE AGED LICENSED NURSING ASSISTANTS.

SONNET IN RED INK- IN SEARCH OF HEALING FROM HIS SISTER'S DEATH, AUTHOR, KETE McCLELLAN CONNECTS WITH LOVE AND THE SPIRIT WORLD.

INDECENT DIANE-BARE SURVIVAL AFTER VERY INDECENT BEHAVIOR. DIANE IS A NEMESIS.

GLITTER'S GRAVEYARD- A TREASURE HUNT ACROSS LATIN AMERICA WITH DIRE RESULTS.

CRIST MISS BLUES- ALCOHOLISM, ADULTERY, ONLINE PRIVACY, AND THE SUPREME COURT WITH SOME HISPANIC LEGEND THROWN IN.

TRACKS OF LOST TEARS-THE SHEDDING OF LIFE'S GREY HUES. BUT IS IT TOO LATE?

SKIN MONSTER-HUMAN TRAFFICKING AT ITS WORST. WILL SHE SURVIVE ITS REACH AND WRATH?

SUNSET OVER THE VILLEROUGE-A CHURCH IN PERIL. LOVER'S SIN AND CORRUPTION. WHO WILL DIE? WHO WILL ESCAPE?

HONOR'S IMPLACABLE SOLDIER – SOLVE CRIME AND SALVE THE MIND TO BRING HEALING TO LIVES HAUNTED BY THE GHOSTS OF DISHONOR AND THE DEATH OF A DAUGHTER DEARLY LOVED

CAPTIVE TO COCOA- THE SAD FACT OF CHILD SLAVERY IN THE CHOCOLATE INDUSTRY

STING OF THE GOLDEN BEE – ENTER THE BEE. MAGIC, MADNESS, AND HISTORY ON THE BRINK EXPLODES BEHIND JEFF'S EYES. HE IS THE ONLY ONE TO SEE.

THE COLOR OF SEIZURES – SUPPORT AND HOPE FOR THOSE WHO ARE CHALLENGED BY PNES.

SEA OF IMPULSE – A SINGER'S WILD LIFE AS REFLECTED THROUGH HER DESCENDENTS TRAVAILS.

SOCK MONKEY LIFE- COLORFUL PHOTOS AND QUIPS ABOUT A VINTAGE SOCK MONKEY.

RULE OF THUMB AND FINGERS- CLEVER AND AMUSING RULES FOR PROPER TEXTING.

ALSO BY JEFFREY UNDERWOOD:

FORBIDDEN TOME-THE TOPSY TURVY LIFE AND TIMES OF HANSEL AND GRETEL AS THEY ESCAPE EVIL CLUTCHES.

LETHAL ASSUMED-THE ARGUMENT FOR THE EXISTENCE OF MONSTERS AND DEMONS IN PRESENT DAY SEATTLE.

ALSO BY KATE TAYLOR:

THE PINK ERASER-FROM TODDLER TO MATURE WOMAN, CODEPENDENT OPAL LEARNS THAT IT IS OKAY TO MAKE MISTAKES.

28945775R00056

Made in the USA
Middletown, DE
01 February 2016